The Creator's Diet

Biblical Insights for Healthy Eating

by

Nicola Burgher

The Creator's

Diet

Biblical Insights for Healthy Eating

by

Nicola Burgher

PNEUMA SPRINGS PUBLISHING UK

Unless otherwise indicated, all Scripture quotations are taken from the New King James Version of the Holy Bible.

First Published 2006
Published by Pneuma Springs Publishing

The Creator's Diet
Copyright © 2006 Nicola Burgher
ISBN10: 0-9545510-8-7
ISBN13: 978-0-954551-08-7

Cover design, editing and typesetting by:
Pneuma Springs Publishing

A Subsidiary of Pneuma Springs Ltd.
230 Lower Road, Belvedere Kent, DA17 6DE.
E: admin@pneumasprings.co.uk
W: www.pneumasprings.co.uk

A catalogue record for this book is available from the British Library.

ACKNOWLEDGEMENTS

To my Mother - the road has not been easy, has it? Who would have thought that you would be both a Mother and Father to me? You have always noted my potential and have been there as a rock through it all. Dad would have been proud. I thank God that you are here to see and read my first publication.

To my brother Marcus—the quiet, super-talented, blessed musician with all the wisdom and knowledge in the world. Thank you for lending me your ear, advising me on the best way to go and encouraging me to launch this publication. I will always maintain that you are the best musician in the world.

To Nicole Berberian, my university buddy! You have been a key figure in my life and an ever-faithful professional support. We've both made it in the media! God has been gracious! Thanks for your time, your professional contribution and your prayers. You look beautiful on that channel five couch! Tell Anoushka and Aren thanks for lending me their mum.

To Dr de Lisser—your input and time has not gone unnoticed. Thank you for everything.

To the team at Pneuma Springs Publishing - in particular the editor; Yomi, many thanks, especially for your patience and encouragement through it all.

And of course my loving Heavenly Father—Jehovah. Praise be to you who has chosen me to do this task and blessed me with the knowledge. Thank you. Your unconditional love surpasses words!

DEDICATION

To my father, the late Reverend Cleveland Samuel Burgher and my eldest brother, Richard Andrew Burgher.

Dad - who passed away on Christmas day, 2004, after being diagnosed with late stage prostate cancer. I saw first-hand the value of nutrition in his life. Good nutrition enabled him to survive longer than the doctor's prognosis, and I in turn had a father for much longer.

Richard - who passed away suddenly on August 26th, 2005 after suffering a suspected asthma attack. I still do not understand.

The two men in my life who demonstrated the true meaning of what it is to be a gentleman, who foresaw my potential and had faith in me. Who were constant inspiration to me and without whom I probably would not have had the motivation or confidence to put into print what you hold in your hands.

I thank God for them. I salute them and dedicate this book to their memories. They will never be forgotten; their legacies will live on in me for as long as I have breath. Thank you for your prayers and your words of encouragement. Thank you for your unconditional love. I love you both. I told you so many times. I meant it. Rest in Peace. Till we meet.

TABLE OF CONTENTS

Chapter I

INTRODUCTION

As Christians we aim to follow Jesus in every area of our lives. However, in reality this is often not the case when it comes to our eating habits.

I have observed that within the church, not much value or place is given to what God says concerning our diet and physical health. In fact, our physical nourishment is one of the areas least talked or preached about. We are quite happy to entrust certain aspects of our lives to God, however when it comes to what we should eat, we gladly take control of this area ourselves, eating whatever we choose, without taking the time to find out what God has to say about it and obey Him. Not many of us realise that Bible-based dietary principles exist, talk less of embracing them in order to nourish our bodies so they can be used effectively to glorify God. God should be glorified in whatever we do, and the Bible is very clear about this;

> *Therefore, whether you eat or drink, or whatever*
> *you do, do all to the glory of God.*
>   1 Corinthians 10:31

For those of us who are aware of the Bible-based principles on diet and health, a large majority do not regard them as being applicable or relevant today. Living in today's fast paced society with a variety of advertising and marketing tactics, targeted at the 'convenience culture', it's all too easy to go for a quick fix when it comes to what we eat. We eat 'convenience' meals in a hurry, believing that we are feeding our bodies properly. A vast majority of us eat primarily for the sake of bridging a hunger gap and give no real thought or consideration to whether we are indeed nourishing our bodies. Sadly, for some of us it is not until we are ill or threatened with illness of some sort that we begin to educate ourselves on healthy eating, make dietary changes for the better, and become careful to feed ourselves with what is nutritionally beneficial.

But whether we realise it or not, or whether we choose to accept it or not, what we put into our body affects us physically, mentally, emotionally and spiritually, consequently affecting how we are able to function. As well as affecting us internally, what we eat will usually affect the way we look on the outside. Thus our eating habits are in a real sense a vital part of our Christian walk.

Of course there are other factors apart from our diet which can influence our level of health, such as our genetic make-up or environmental factors such as exposure to viruses, toxins, pollution. However a poor diet is a primary cause of many of the illnesses we are familiar with today, and this combined with genetic and environmental factors will only further increase our risk of ill health.

Jesus cares about our health. Our health is as important to Him now as it was back then, when He physically walked the earth and healed the sick. It is His desire for us to be whole and this includes wholeness in body as well as mind and spirit. He is our Creator, and no one knows better than Him, how best we can nourish the body He has given to us.

Most of us lack the fundamental knowledge of what our bodies require to operate efficiently. The Bible says;

> *My people are destroyed for lack of knowledge.*
>
> Hosea 4:6

The neglect and ignorance of this important area has put us, and will continue to put us at greater risk of ill health, and for some, even premature death.

As a result of this apparent lack of dietary knowledge in the 'body of Christ', I feel burdened to write and highlight Bible-based nutritional principles in order to reduce our risk of ill health and disease. I believe that when we take the time to become educated in the area

13

of nutrition and health, we will be better equipped to make the right dietary choices, as well as take positive steps to improve our health and overall well-being.

We can be absolutely certain that our Creator would not give us instructions on every area of our life and somehow forget to include how we should take care of our physical nourishment! We need to acknowledge what He says concerning every area of our lives – including our eating habits. God has made provision for us in His Word, and we can be sure that what God instructs us to do is always for our good. His word says;

> *For I know the thoughts I think towards you,*
> *says the Lord, thoughts of peace and not of evil,*
> *to give you a future and a hope.*
>
> Jeremiah 29:11

Our lives are too precious to the Lord to be wasted on days, months or years of unnecessary and preventable ill health. God designed true living on earth to be one of divine health, joy, ecstasy, vitality, abundance and purpose, and He has placed a certain level of responsibility on us to maintain – as much as possible – our health and well-being.

God wants us to be whole and prosperous in every area of our lives. Believe it or not, He is as interested in our physical wholeness, as He is in every other area of our lives. God has a passion to see us whole.

It is impossible to include absolutely everything on nutrition in one single book. Besides, in my experience, giving too much information at once can sometimes be confusing and off-putting. Therefore as we go through the pages of this book we will explore Biblical dietary principles and learn what kinds of foods God views as suitable for consumption. We will also examine the nutritional benefits of various foods essential for a healthy diet, with the aim of helping you to make the right dietary choices based on tested and tried principles of God's eternal word.

May God bless you as you read and digest the message He has placed on my heart to deliver to you.

Chapter II

GOD'S VIEWS ON FOOD

God in His infinite wisdom has not only made provision for us but has also left us with a detailed manual – His own Word – to help us through this life and remind us of the rewards in the next. Throughout the Bible, God gives us instructions and guidance on just about everything we need to know – from good hygiene practices to safe sexual practices and moral conduct. Also contained within the Bible are instructions, principles and promises on how we are to take care of ourselves physically, including what to put into our bodies to help maintain health and well-being.

Our body is referred to as God's Temple,

> *Or do you not know that your body is a temple of the Holy Spirit, who is in you, whom you have from God and you are not your own? For you were bought at a price; therefore glorify God in your body and in your spirit which are God's.*
>
> 1 Corinthians 6:19, 20

The Bible says we should take care of the temple, not only from a spiritual perspective but equally from a physical one. Thankfully, it's not up to us to decide what is best for optimum care and peak performance of our temple.

So, let's take a look at God's principles governing food. For some of us, this may be the first time we have considered what God has to say about diet. We need to study in order to benefit from the gems of wisdom and knowledge God has freely given us. The Bible has this to say about our responsibility to study;

> *Be diligent to present yourself approved to God, a worker who does not need to be ashamed, rightly dividing the word of truth.*
>
> 2 Timothy 2:15

The Bible-based dietary principles mentioned here are relevant for our health today and will be covered in detail in later chapters. These principles have no application to the salvation of the soul but are primarily for the benefit of the body. Applying them will help us greatly reduce the risk of ill health. They are listed below in no particular order:

Principle #1 – The prohibition of fat

> *This shall be a perpetual statute throughout your generations in all your dwellings: you shall eat neither fat nor blood.*
>
> Leviticus 3:17

> *Speak to the children of Israel saying you shall not eat any fat of ox or sheep or goat. And the fat of an animal that dies naturally, and the fat of what is torn by wild beasts may be used in any other way but you shall by no means eat it.*
>
> Leviticus 7:23-24

The fat forbidden in the Scriptures above refers to the hard cover fat of animals and not the internal marbling fat of the flesh we eat when we cook meat. Fat that covers the internal organs should be avoided as well.

Fat is a tissue in the body that stores energy. Unfortunately, animal fat or saturated fat as it is also referred to, can store harmful chemicals e.g. herbicides, antibiotics, hormones, insecticides. It is a fact that the over-consumption of hard fat, or saturated fat (fat that is firmest at room temperature) is associated with increased incidences of certain cancers, heart disease and obesity. It appears that God, in His wisdom was protecting us from harm and ill health, when He forbade the eating of fat.

Principle #2 – Harmful and Healthful Meats

> *...that you may distinguish between the holy and the unholy, and between the unclean and the*

clean.

Leviticus 10:10

After the flood, meats were introduced into the diet. For whatever reason, God later declared certain meats as fit for consumption and others unfit; these will be discussed in more detail in a later chapter where I will show that the meats forbidden in Leviticus are actually not as nourishing as the ones God recommends for consumption. This principle is a little harder for us to apply, as we cannot fully understand why we shouldn't eat certain meats – particularly as it concerns Old Testament Law, and more importantly to us, if they taste nice!

Principle #3 - The prohibition of blood

> *But you shall not eat flesh with its life, that is, it's blood.*
>
> Genesis 9:4

> *However, you may slaughter and eat meat within all your gates......only you shall not eat the blood; you shall pour it on the earth like water.*
>
> Deuteronomy 12:15-16

> *Only be sure that you do not eat the blood, for the blood is the life. You may not eat the life with the meat. You shall not eat it; you shall pour it on the earth like water.*
>
> Deuteronomy 12:23-24

Other biblical references for the prohibition of blood can be found in Leviticus 3:17, 7:26,27, 19:26, 1 Samuel

14:32-34

This principle is one of the easier principles for us to adhere to; after all, no one in their right mind really wants to dine on a serving of blood? For us the thought of it is quite repulsive and thus we logically find this principle very easy to apply.

The Bible says that the blood is "the life". Thus eating the blood could be seen as disrespect for life. Similarly, from the first shedding of blood for the covering of Adam and Eve's nakedness in the Garden of Eden to the shedding of Christ's blood on the cross for the atonement of the sins of mankind, blood is given much significance. Thus blood has its purpose and function within a biblical context; therefore it is not to be consumed as food or drink.

Some Bible scholars have attributed the prohibition of blood as a protective measure given by God to His people due to the blood's natural function of transporting waste materials for elimination by the body. The logic here is that by forbidding the consumption of blood, God is protecting his people from consuming unhealthy waste material, and potential ill health.

We could speculate about why God chose to prohibit the consumption of blood, but we may never really know the reason(s) unless He chooses to reveal it to us. Whatever the case, our part is not to speculate or debate. God is all-wise and therefore must have good reasons for whatever He does or says. Let us simply trust and obey Him.

About the Bible-based Dietary Principles

Although the three principles above are connected with an element of uncleanness or cleanness, holiness or unholiness they are also connected with what is harmful or healthful to eat. We must simply trust God concerning what He has declared to be healthy or unfit for our consumption.

Even though we are in the world, we are not of the world; we have become new creatures - people who do not do things the world's way but God's way. Our behaviour, our attitude, our thoughts, even our eating habits must differ from the world's and should reflect Christ in us.

God knows that whatever we put into His Temple - our body - could affect us for the better or for the worse. The choice of foods we eat will affect our:

- Mental performance (e.g. our concentration, clarity and sharpness of mind)..
- physical performance (our energy levels).
- emotional status and balance.
- our level of disease and infection (resistance and protection).
- and can ultimately affect our quality of life and overall lifespan - all of which directly affect our spiritual performance and the level at which we can effectively serve God.

In the remaining sections of this chapter we shall contrast God's dietary principles with the world's dietary principles. This will enable us to better understand God's stipulations concerning what we should eat.

God's Versus The World's Dietary Principles

Many times, in our own wisdom, we think we know what is best for us. In our own eyes we may think we are eating healthily, however in reality this may not be the case. As a result of our ignorance we do more harm than good in the long run, and we regret our actions. Often after things have not worked out the way we think they should, we realise that we were wrong and then turn to God to find out His way of doing things. The Bible states;

> *There is a way that seems right to a man but its end is the way of death.*
>
> Proverbs 14:12

> *Do not be wise in your own eyes; fear the Lord and depart from evil. It will be health to your flesh and strength to your bones.*
>
> Proverbs 3:7,8

God is the authority on everything we need to know including nutrition. If we briefly compare His dietary principles and the world's dietary principles, we will see that God's way is far superior, trustworthy and beneficial for us.

God's Dietary Principles

- Controlled and instructed by our loving Creator and Father.
- Simple, cost effective, medically proven and sensible.
- Consistent and enduring.
- Based on healthy, healing foods.
- Based on natural foods that the body was designed to process, in the right quantities.
- Low in harmful fats, rich in natural good fats, high in fibre, low in cholesterol.
- Rich in vitamins, minerals and trace elements essential for bodily function.
- Contain a good balance of proteins, water, natural sugars, fats and healing protective substances - called antioxidants and phytonutrients.
- Created with our best interests as a priority.

**Results:** Optimal nutrition and diminished risk of ill health. If adhered to, God's principles on diet will lead us into a nutritious eating plan that ministers health and healing, simultaneously. We will be more likely to have a healthy body, mind and spirit that function for what they were originally created to do – to glorify the Creator.

The World's Dietary Principles

- Controlled by man; the media, the government and

various other man-orientated influences.

- Confusing, expensive and unwise.
- Subject to various influences, change and variation
- Made up of 'convenience', highly processed items containing numerous substances our body was not designed to process such as additives, artificial colours, artificial ingredients and harmful chemicals.
- Food components that are high in fat, sugar, and salt.
- Low in vitamins, minerals and essential nutrients.
- Not necessarily created with our best interests as a priority – monetary gain and profit is more of a priority.

Results: An increased risk of ill health potentially leading to some of the dietary related illnesses we are familiar with, for example hypertension (high blood pressure), obesity, lethargy (extreme tiredness all the time), irritability, behavioural problems, certain cancers, addictions, tooth decay, anaemias, hormone imbalances e.g. diabetes, thyroid, mental health problems, constipation, heart disease, gallstones, kidney failure, indigestion, ulcers etc

Chapter III

THE CREATOR'S DIET: PLANT FOODS

And God said, See I have given you every herb that yields seed which is on the face of all the earth.

Genesis 1:29a

This instruction includes many plants and their products like wheat, oats, rice, barley, millet, rye and other grains also referred to as starchy carbohydrates, legumes (peas, beans and lentils), bush and vine-bearing fruits and vegetables (melons, grapes, berries, squash, tomatoes, cucumber, egg plant etc.)

...and every tree whose fruit yields seed; to you it shall be for food.

Genesis 1:29b

This instruction includes all fruit as well as nuts.

Then in Genesis 3, after Adam and Eve sinned in the Garden of Eden, God instructed

...And you shall eat the herb of the field.

Genesis 3:18b

This includes herbs without seed in them such as lettuce, broccoli, cabbage, cauliflower, spinach, asparagus, and tubers – (yams, potatoes, carrots, beets etc).

Thus God's instructions give us liberty to eat foods from the plant kingdom i.e. starchy carbohydrates, fruits and vegetables (including nuts and seeds).

Let's look at these food classifications in a little more detail.

Carbohydrates
Carbohydrates are the preferred source of energy or fuel for the body and provide us with vitamins, minerals and fibre. Current advice from nutritionists recommend that at least 50% of our dietary energy intake or a third of our dietary intake should come from 'carbohydrate-rich' foods such as bread, rice, flour products, yams, cassava, green bananas, potatoes (including sweet potatoes) and squashes, plantains, pastas and noodles, cereals like oats and barley, millet,

maize, quinoa and cornmeal. Amazing isn't it, that God knew this before nutritionists started recommending it as a healthy way of eating!

The Brown Foods

Brown or wholegrain rice, bread and pasta contain more goodness in the form of vitamins and minerals and fibre than their white counterparts. Fibre helps to keep our digestive system healthy by reducing the risk of constipation – a risk factor for bowel cancer. Wholemeal bread is more nutritious than white bread as it is made using all three parts of a grain of wheat – the endosperm, the wheatgerm and the bran. As a result, it has much more nutrients than you would find in white bread which is made with the least nutritious part of the grain – the endosperm. Because wholemeal bread has more fibre, it also keeps you feeling fuller for longer. Look out for foods that contain 6g fibre per 100g of food. These foods are termed high fibre foods and are very good for you. Start introducing brown foods into your daily diet from today.

Fruits and Vegetables

Fruits and vegetables come under the bracket of carbohydrates. Current advice from nutritionists tell us how important fruit and vegetable consumption is and recommends that we aim to eat at least five portions of fruit and vegetables a day.

Consuming fruit and vegetables is very important. By eating a variety of fruit and vegetables regularly and consistently we provide our bodies with a power-house of nourishment essential for health. Consumption of fruits and vegetables is encouraged because they are excellent sources of vitamins, minerals and trace elements. It is interesting that nutritionists are now emphasizing the importance of eating fruit and vegetables. God recommended eating fruit and vegetables since the beginning of time; before nutritionists and health professionals started advertising, it was already there in His Word!

What exactly is a portion of fruit and vegetables?
Current recommendations are to consume at least five portions of fruit and vegetables a day which can mean 2 portions of fruit and 3 portions of vegetables, or 3 portions of fruit and 2 portions of vegetables – as long as the portions add up to at least 5 portions a day, you are on the right track. To help you consume your daily portions of fruit and vegetables, remember that one portion is equivalent to:

- ½ a large fruit such as mango, papaya or grapefruit.
- 1 medium fruit such as an apple, orange, banana, peach or pear.
- 2 small fruits such as satsumas, apricots, plums or kiwi fruits
- 1 glass of fruit juice (preferably freshly squeezed or blended).
- 2-3 tablespoons of cooked vegetables such as broccoli, cauliflower, carrots and green beans
- 1 small bowl of salad.
- Matchbox size portion of raisins.

Consuming more than 5 portions a day is allowed and highly recommended. Start eating a variety of fruits and vegetables today!

No Cheating!
Fruit juices, vegetable and fruit smoothies, baked beans and pulses only count as ONE portion no matter how much you consume in one day!

To help increase your daily fruit and vegetable consumption, why not try snacking on fruit instead of chocolate, crisps and cakes when hungry, or try adding dried or fresh fruit to breakfast cereals, having a salad with lunch or main meals or adding salad to a sandwich? Adding more vegetables to casseroles or soups is also another good habit to form, or having a glass of freshly squeezed fruit juice at breakfast, or fruit for dessert instead of those soggy puddings? And remember, it is important that we eat a variety of fruit and vegetables to get a good combination of the nutrients the body can use on a daily basis.

What are vitamins, minerals and trace elements and how do they help us?

Vitamins are needed by our bodies in small amounts and are essential for the body's effective functioning. Vitamins are generally divided into two categories - fat soluble vitamins (vitamins A, D, E and K) and water soluble vitamins (thiamine [B1]), riboflavin [B2], niacin

[B3], pantothenic acid, biotin, folate [folic acid], vitamin B6, vitamin B12 and vitamin C). The body doesn't need fat-soluble vitamins every day as they are stored by the liver for when they are needed. Fat-soluble vitamins are found in foods such as butter, vegetable oils, dairy foods and oily fish. Water-soluble vitamins on the other hand are not stored by the body and are therefore needed more frequently. If we have more than we need, the body gets rid of them when we urinate. Water-soluble vitamins are found in fruits and vegetables. They can also be found in starchy carbohydrates like oats and barley, millet, maize, quinoa. Our body needs both the fat-soluble vitamins and water-soluble vitamins to operate properly.

Minerals and trace elements

Minerals, like vitamins, are needed by the body in small or trace amounts and are important for effective bodily function. As well as fruit and vegetables, minerals are also found in meat, cereal products such as bread, fish, milk and dairy foods and nuts. Calcium, iron, magnesium, phosphorus, potassium, sodium and sulphur are all essential minerals needed by the body. Trace elements are essential for the body to function effectively and are needed in even smaller amounts than vitamins and minerals. Trace elements are also found in meat, cereal products, fish, dairy foods and nuts.

Each vitamin, mineral and trace element has its very own function in the body and this is the reason each vitamin is as important as the next. The table in Appendix I summarises the functions of the essential vitamins, minerals and trace elements for you at a glance.

Immune-boosting power of vitamins and minerals

Some vitamins, minerals and trace elements help the functioning of our immune system. Vitamin A, B1, B2, B6, B12, folate, vitamin C, vitamin E, iron, zinc, magnesium and selenium are all involved in the functioning of our immune system. Fruits and vegetables are excellent sources of these nutrients – especially oranges, kiwi fruits, watermelons, berries, carrots, beetroots, sweet potatoes, tomatoes, sweet peppers, bean sprouts.

Boost your body's natural defence

Our immune system is our body's natural defence mechanism that identifies anything unfamiliar and removes it. Its role is to protect the body from harmful invaders, thus keeping it in as good condition as possible. Eating a diet rich in fruits and vegetables is important for the effective functioning of your immune system. Eat a mixture of raw and cooked fruit and vegetables, as some nutrients can be destroyed during preparation and cooking.

As well as providing the body with vitamins and minerals, fruits and vegetables are excellent sources of;

- Carotenes – yellow or orange-red pigments in

plants which give them their characteristic colour. Carotenes are necessary for growth and development and have been associated with the prevention of certain cancers, heart disease and resistance to infection. It is thus very important to eat red, yellow and orange foods as these are rich in carotenes e.g. carrots, tomatoes, apricots, sweet potatoes, squashes, watermelons, papaya, oranges, sweet peppers etc.

- Phytonutrients - include carotenes and have beneficial effects on health by helping to protect against a number of diseases such as heart disease and cancer. Appendix II summarises some phytonutrients and their functions in the body.

- Fibre - helps to keep the digestive system healthy and helps to prevent digestive disorders such as constipation and bowel cancer.

- Carbohydrate –a source of energy for the body

- Water – the main ingredient in all the fluids that make up our body systems e.g. the blood, our digestive juices. Water is also needed for the transport of nutrients to our cells, of waste products from our cells and organs out of the body and for hydration of body cells.

- Antioxidants – reduce the effects of harmful substances responsible for cancers and ageing that may enter the body through what we eat or breathe in.

> **God's added protection**
> I like to refer to fruits and vegetables as God's super foods. Fruits and vegetables are excellent sources of phytonutrients and antioxidants. A diet rich in fruit and vegetables helps to prevent disease and promote health at the same time. Phytonutrients are as important as vitamins and minerals to our health. They are not stored in our body therefore it is important to consume them regularly to get the full benefits. Phytonutrient activity has been associated with boosting immune function, anti cancer activity, antibiotic activity, protection against varicose veins, bleeding gums, menopausal activities, fibroids and other hormone-related diseases to name a few. So eat up your fruits and vegetables!

It is important to eat a variety of fruits and vegetables on a daily basis. Fresh, frozen, dried and canned fruit and vegetables all count towards our daily intake of fruit and vegetables.

Nuts and seeds

> *And God said, See I have given you every herb that yields seed which is on the face of all the earth, and every tree whose fruit yields seed; to you it shall be for food.*
>
> Genesis 1:29

God has given us freedom to eat nuts and seeds. Like carbohydrates, His directive for us to eat nuts and seeds was one of His first instructions. Nuts, like seeds are part of the grain family. If we choose to consume nuts and seeds, we should really only consume them in moderate amounts, as they can be high in fat and overall calories, if eaten in excess.

Nuts about Nuts and Seeds

Nuts and seeds are part of the grain family. Although they can be high in fat and calories, the fats are good fats that help repair damaged cells in the body. They are also a very good source of vitamins and protein. Eat them in moderation and in their raw form; not processed or covered in sugar, salt and oil!

Our body was specifically designed to run on food from the plant kingdom (carbohydrates, fruits and vegetables, nuts and seeds) because these foods:

- Contain good natural fats that our body was designed to process.

- Are excellent sources of natural fibre needed to help maintain a healthy digestive system.

- Are excellent sources of vitamins and minerals needed by the body on a daily basis to perform a variety of important functions.

- Contain the right balance of protein, water and natural sugars.

- Contain special substances known as anti-oxidants and phytonutrients which work to protect the body from disease and harmful substances.

- And above all, our loving Father says they are good for food.

Remember to eat a variety of these foods. No one food will provide us with all the nutrition our body needs.

Be adventurous and experiment. Try new dishes, new ideas, and new cooking methods. You can make healthy eating fun - for you, your family and friends.

Chapter IV

THE CREATOR'S DIET: ANIMAL FOODS

Meats are a source of protein, vitamins and minerals such as iron, zinc, vitamin B6 and vitamin B12. Fish is also a source of protein and good fats needed for a whole host of bodily functions. After the flood, God introduced meat into the diet,

> *So God blessed Noah and His sons and said to them "Be fruitful and multiply and fill the earth. And the fear of you and the dread of you shall be on every beast of the earth, on every bird of the air, on all that move on the earth, and on all the fish of the sea. They are given into your hand.*

39

Every moving thing that lives shall be food for you.

Genesis 9:1-3a

However, later in Leviticus, God separates those animals into two categories; those which are good to eat and those which are not. Appendix III summarises those animals which God deems fit and unfit to eat, as is evident in the Scriptures below:

Among the animals, whatever divides the hoof, having cloven hooves and chewing the cud – that you may eat.

Leviticus 11:3,

These you may eat of all that are in the water; whatever in the water that has fins and scales. Whatever in the seas or in the rivers – that you may eat.

Leviticus 11:9

And these you shall regard as an abomination among the birds, they shall not be eaten, they are an abomination; the eagle, the vulture, the buzzard, the kite and the falcon after its kind, the ostrich, the short-eared owl, the seagull and the hawk after its kind, the little owl, the fisher owl, and the screech owl, the white owl, the jackdaw, and the carrion vulture, the stork, the heron after its kind, the hoopoe and the bat, all flying insects that creep on all fours shall be an abomination to you.

Leviticus 11:13-20

Animals good for food

We have seen that the Bible considers some animals as healthy for consumption and others, unhealthy. Understandably for many, this principle might be a little difficult to accept and even harder to apply especially if we have been eating those animals that are not considered good for food. And it will be harder still if they taste delicious and we see them as doing us no harm. However, God's thoughts and ways are higher than ours – and sometimes we cannot begin to understand why He says and does some things. All we know is that He knows the end from the beginning - the bigger picture - and our duty is to trust His wisdom and sound judgement. If He says it, we are to believe by faith that there is a good reason for it! After all, we do believe He loves us.

From a purely nutritional standpoint, animals which the Lord says are good for food 'co-incidentally' have very effective digestive systems. A good digestive system means that the maximum goodness from the food is absorbed and waste products are eliminated effectively. This means when we eat the flesh of these animals, we are eating wholesome meat. Secondly, the diets of these animals are based primarily on healthful substances such as grains and grasses so we have added protection. This suggests that God in His wisdom had taken into consideration our nutritional needs, long before we were born. He really does look after His creation – you and me – just to ensure that we get the best in life.

Animals not good for food

Animals stated as unhealthy to eat are generally gluttonous. Gluttony does not simply mean; "to overeat" but also implies the consumption of everything and anything (good or bad)! Because of this, these animals are more likely to be vehicles of transmission for harmful diseases. Some of the animals in this list are termed "scavengers", because of their primary role in cleaning up the earth and purifying in the sea. Eating these kinds of animals and their contents has implications for our health in both the short and long-term. Our body is the temple of the living God so we really should not be putting everything and anything into it.

> *Or do you not know that your body is the temple of the Holy Spirit, who is in you, whom you have from God, and you are not your own.*
>
> 1 Corinthians 6:19

Consumption of these meats can prove detrimental to our health by introducing into our bodies "slow toxins" in the form of parasites, bacteria and/or viruses.

Not everything that looks like food, smells good and tastes good is necessarily nourishing or fit for consumption. Thankfully our loving Father has outlined those foods that are good to eat and those which are not. Rather than playing "Russian roulette" with our eating habits, let us trust that our Father really knows what is best for us.

Is Clean and Unclean Relevant for Today?

A comment I hear time and time again when discussing clean and unclean meats in the Bible is that God's instructions concerning these were under the Law, and thus is no more applicable to us now that we are under grace.

One of the Scriptures quoted to support this view is 1 Timothy 4:4 which states;

> *For every creature of God is good, and nothing is to be refused if it is received with thanksgiving, for it is sanctified by the Word of God and prayer.*

1 Timothy 4:4

When interpreting Scripture, it is crucial that we put into context what is being said—firstly, relative to the religious culture of the time and secondly from the perspective, beliefs and culture of the one speaking.

In the above scripture, Paul writes a letter to Timothy. Being a Jew, when he refers to creatures that are good for food, he is of course referring to those which God calls food (Appendix III). Paul would not be referring to those creatures God had said should not be consumed. In practical terms, it would be a wrong application of Scripture to consume unhealthy or 'junk food' continually and say it is okay because we have sanctified it with the word of God and prayer!

Another point commonly raised is that the dietary laws were given as a ceremonial act of sanctification and are no longer applicable today. Indeed it is true that the death of Jesus Christ and the shedding of His blood

43

removed the need for ceremonial regulations. However, what we fail to realise is that within these Bible-based dietary principles are protection, health and life and the only way we can reap the benefits is to embrace the principles and live in obedience to them. Though the ceremonial side of these principles may no longer be necessary, we can definitely benefit physically from applying the laws.

On a practical note, I recommend eating red meat no more than twice a week at the most as red meat contains higher levels of saturated fat than white meat or fish. Our meals should be centred around the carbohydrates.

A Word About Meats

Meats and poultry are optional and are not a necessity in the diet i.e. you can live without them. Our bodies do not need huge amounts of protein, as they were not designed to process huge amounts of protein. Meats do provide a good source of protein, however they should be eaten in moderation as they can be high in saturated fat which is associated with obesity, heart disease and certain cancers. Consider meats and poultry to be celebration or luxury foods rather than everyday foods. And where possible, purchase organic, kosher (well slaughtered and prepared) meats and fish.

In terms of everyday portions, a good rule is to have one half the plate full of vegetables, one quarter of starch e.g. rice or potatoes or pasta, and the rest protein e.g. meat or vegetarian alternatives.

In fact, you don't have to eat meat to survive, but if you do, ensure that it is meat good for food and where possible, free-range, organic meat.

A Word About Fish

Oily fish are very important in your diet. Eating oily fish such as herring, mackerel, trout, tuna (fresh, not tinned), salmon, sardines, pilchards can help to control cholesterol levels, enhance brain function and vision, learning ability, co-ordination and mood. They are also associated with improved immune function and metabolism, reduced inflammation and maintenance of water balance. The Government currently recommends that we eat at least two portions of fish a week, one of which should be oily fish.

Is healthful meat safe today? - Going Organic!

Unfortunately these days, animals for food are not reared the same way as they were in biblical times. For a start many are kept cooped up in refined, over-crowded places, and are slaughtered differently causing them to release hormones and chemicals at the time of slaughter. Similarly many are given large doses of pesticides, antibiotics, hormone residues, food additives, artificial fertilisers and chemical additives. Whilst they have their purpose, regular consumption of these chemicals can stop nutrients from being absorbed and used by our bodies, and in some instances can promote the excretion of valuable vitamins and minerals. Indeed, an over-load of these substances in our body can exceed its capacity to detoxify itself, resulting in some of the diseases and disorders discussed earlier, plus others we may not currently be aware of.

The word 'organic' is defined by the law. Any food labelled organic must meet a set of strict standards, some of which include:

- Restricting the use of artificial chemical fertilizers and pesticides.
- Relying on developing healthy fertile soil and growing a mixture of crops.
- Rearing animals without routine use of drugs and antibiotics.

Organic food production is based on a system of farming that maintains and replenishes soil fertility without the use of toxic pesticides and fertilizers. Organic foods are minimally processed without artificial ingredients, preservatives, or irradiation to maintain the integrity of food. In fact, although it is now impossible to totally avoid man-made chemicals, choosing organic foods is the nearest we can get to eating a pure diet and reducing the risk of an over-load of these chemicals in our bodies.

Any organic product sold in the UK must by law display a certification symbol or number. When you see an organic symbol, it means the product complies with minimum government standards. The Soil Association organic symbol is the UK's main certification mark.

Organic Issues

If you cannot afford to purchase organic produce, don't despair. At the very least you should wash and peel your vegetables and fruits, and try and purchase free-range products. There is no conclusive evidence that organic produce is better, nutritionally, however by going organic, you will be reducing the levels of toxins you put into your body.

What about eggs?

Eggs are similar to meat because, like meat, they are a good source of protein. Eat eggs only from those animals God has said are good to eat i.e. chickens, and hens etc. And go for free-range where possible. Mind you, eggs, like meat should be eaten as a luxury or celebration food. Your diet is to be based around foods from the plant kingdom.

Vegetarianism

Though there is nothing wrong with eating meat the argument that meat must be consumed to obtain all the nutrients the body needs is untrue. There is no nutrient (with the exception of vitamin B12) that cannot be obtained in products from the plant kingdom. In fact, research has shown that the vegetarian diet is healthier than the typical meat-eater's diet. Biblically, the initial diet given by God was vegetarian and the life span of those who ate it came close to 1000 years!

More and more individuals are turning to vegetarianism. Restaurants are now offering more vegetarian options, even though at times it can still be difficult to eat out as a vegetarian or vegan.

There are three main types of vegetarians:

- The lacto-ovovegetarian who consumes eggs, milk and milk products.
- The lacto-vegetarian who consumes no eggs but milk and milk products.
- The vegan who consumes no animal products whatsoever.

Although being a vegetarian or vegan is a healthy way to eat, both have to be careful to adhere to eating a healthy, balanced diet. Indeed, vegans in particular have to be especially careful that they are consuming a nutritionally adequate diet.

Vegans should be particularly careful to consume enough of the following vitamins and minerals:

- Calcium – obtained from dark green leafy vegetables such as watercress, kale and cauliflower also soybeans, sesame seeds, dried fruit, citrus fruits, and black strap molasses.
- Riboflavin[B2]– found in green leafy vegetables, mushrooms, squashes and almonds.
- Vitamin D – made by the act of sunlight on the skin for 15-20 minutes and also found in soy milk.
- Zinc – found in legumes, whole grains and wheatgerm.
- Iron – found in legumes, dried fruit, green leafy vegetables and whole grains. The absorption of iron is enhanced by the consumption of vitamin C

which is found in a wide variety of fruit and vegetables such as peppers, broccoli, oranges and kiwi fruit, sweet potatoes, brussel sprouts.

- Vitamin B12 – even though we only need tiny amounts of this vitamin, it is not found in any plant sources. In fact, it is largely found in meat and eggs. It may be advisable for vegans to take a supplement of vitamin B12. Alternatively, vitamin B12 is found in fortified breakfast cereals, veggie burgers, fortified soy milk and fermented soybean (miso).

For more information on vegetarianism and vegetarian diets, visit the Vegetarian Society by logging on to www.vegsoc.org or call 0161 925 2000.

Alternatives to Meats and Fish

Soya, nuts, seeds, mycoprotein, Texturized Vegetable Protein (TVP), beans (e.g. kidney beans, baked beans) and pulses provide a source of protein, vitamins and minerals for those of us who do not eat meat or fish. In fact, foods from the plant kingdom will also provide adequate protein, natural fats, fibre, water, vitamins and minerals.

Milk and dairy products

Milk and dairy products include foods such as milks, cheeses, and yogurts. Since milk could not be stored in biblical times, it was fermented to keep it from spoiling. The cheese, butter and yogurt mentioned in the Bible are referred to as 'curds' and are thus healthful for us to eat. Soya alternatives can also be included as they are fortified with calcium.

Like meat and eggs, milk and dairy products are not essential to have in the diet i.e. we can live without them. The initial diet prescribed by God did not have dairy products or milk. However, if we do choose to eat them, we should eat them in moderation, as they contain saturated fats - of which an increased consumption is associated with increased risk of obesity, heart disease and certain cancers.

An Important Principle to Remember
As much as possible, try to eat foods in their natural form – i.e. the way they were originally created, before they were changed or converted into something else that humans think is better for us. Try unflavoured, no added sugar bio-yogurts (live yogurts) and sweeten them yourself.

Remember that our diet should focus around the plant kingdom (carbohydrates, fruits and vegetables, nuts and seeds), which will provide our bodies with a blend of essential nutrients needed for effective functioning. When eaten in moderation, milk and dairy products provide us with a good balance of protein, some vitamins and minerals such as vitamin A, vitamin B12 and vitamin B2. One serving of dairy food is equal to one small pot of yogurt [150g], or one piece of cheese (matchbox size), or a small glass of milk. Current recommendations for dairy products is not to eat more than two to three servings a day.

Chapter V

FATTY AND SUGARY FOODS

Fat is naturally present in certain foods items such as nuts, seeds, fruits, vegetables and legumes, milk and dairy products, fish and meat. Pure butter and unrefined/unprocessed oils like extra virgin olive oil are also included in this grouping.

However, as discussed earlier, there are specific instructions in the Bible with regards to the consumption of fat, and scientists are now confirming this age-old message given by God thousands of years ago.

Our bodies are not designed to process large amounts of fat or sugar and other items which are rich in these

51

components; for example, margarines, fat spreads, cooking oils, salad dressings, mayonnaise, cream, fried foods, chocolate, crisps, biscuits, pastries, cakes, puddings, ice-creams, rich sauces/gravies, soft drinks and fizzy drinks, sweets, sugar coated breakfast cereals, jam, sugar etc. These foods not only contain high amounts of fat and/or sugar, but are subject to a level of processing that negatively affects their nutritional profile.

Consuming foods rich in saturated fat has been associated with raised cholesterol levels and blood pressure, an increased risk of certain cancers, obesity and heart disease. Our body does need fat but they must be the right kinds. Unfortunately we are consuming too much of the wrong kinds of fats – saturated fat – found in all fats of animal origin including dairy items such as whole milk, cream, cheese, fatty meats such as beef, veal, lamb and meat pies, and processed convenience food often referred to as "junk-food", and not enough of the essential fats such as omega 3 found in oily fish, green leafy vegetables, Soya and seeds e.g. sunflower, sesame, flaxseeds. And as fat is very addictive, the more we continue to eat the more of it we want to eat.

What about hydrogenated fats and trans fatty acids?

Hydrogenation is a form of processing used to turn liquid oils into solid fat. This results in hydrogenated vegetable oils, or hydrogenated fats. Hydrogenated fats are used in some biscuits, cakes, pastries, margarines, vegetable shortenings and other processed foods.

During the hydrogenation process, substances called trans fatty acids may be formed. These fats have no known nutritional benefits. In fact they do more harm than good by raising the type of cholesterol in the blood that increases the risk of coronary heart disease. It is thought that the action of trans fatty acids is worse than that of saturated fat!

So as part of a healthy eating plan we should reduce the consumption of foods containing these artificial fats. In fact, we should try and reduce the amount of total fat in our diet by consuming a greater proportion of fruits, vegetables and starchy carbohydrates.

Natural Trans fats

Natural trans fatty acids are found in very low doses in foods such as dairy products, meat and lamb. Because they are found naturally and at very low levels they present no harm to us. Also if these foods are eaten in their correct proportions we really have nothing to worry about.

Refined sugar

Refined sugar is found in high amounts in processed products such as jams, preserves, biscuits, cakes, pies, pastries, donuts, milkshakes, canned fruits, fruit juices, sweets, chocolate, confectionery, some breakfast cereals, fizzy drinks etc. Some fizzy drinks can contain in excess of six teaspoons of sugar! These foods offer little or no real nutritional value, and due to their addictive nature, can lead to health issues such as obesity, tooth decay, irritability, lethargy, behavioural problems, addictions, hormone imbalance disorders such as diabetes and other long-term health problems.

Food labels

To help us avoid foods high in fat and sugar, it's important that we read and understand food labels. The Government is finally clamping down on the advertising of items that are high in fat and sugar and current guidelines are as follows:

- 20g of fat (or more) per 100g of food is considered high in fat. 5g of saturated fat (or more) is also considered high in fat.

- 3g of fat (or less) per 100g of food is considered low fat. 1g of saturated fat (or less) per 100g is also considered low fat.

- 10g of sugar (or more) per 100g of food is considered high in sugar. (Look for the carbohydrates (of which sugars) figure).

- 2g of sugar (or less) per 100g of food is considered low in sugar.

If our diets are based around the starchy carbohydrates and also rich in fruit and vegetables, not only will we be consuming foods that are healthy and nutritious, but also foods that contain natural sugars and fats in the correct proportions hence we reduce our risk of various diseases common today. At the same time, we will be eating foods which are satisfying and therefore we will be less likely to snack on foods high in fat and sugar.

If you truly cannot avoid products high in fat and sugar, eat them very, very sparingly.

A Word on Salt/Sodium

Foods that are high in sugar and fat may also be high in salt. Eating too much salt is associated with raised blood pressure and thus an increased risk of stroke and heart disease. In fact, people with high blood pressure are three times as likely to have a stroke or develop heart disease than people with normal blood pressure.

Many of us don't think we eat a lot of salt because we don't add it to food; however the majority of salt in the diet – 75% - comes from the salt present in processed foods such as bread, some breakfast cereals, soups, sauces, meat and meat products, ready meals and food items, confectionery, some biscuits, cakes and some seasonings.

Salt or Sodium?

Salt is made up of sodium and chloride and it's the sodium that is associated with raising the blood pressure and increasing the risk of heart disease and stroke. In order to convert sodium to salt, multiply the sodium by 2.5!

Current recommendations encourage us to reduce the amount of salt we consume. In general, we should really have no more than 6g of salt per day or 2.5g of sodium. In practical terms this means eating less processed foods and not adding salt during preparation, but using alternative seasonings such as apple cider vinegar, onions, challots, garlic, chillies and peppers, lime, lemon juices, and other herbs and spices. Although it may not taste the same, it's definitely better for your health and after a while your taste will surprisingly adapt to a lower salt diet.

To help us identify foods that are high in salt/sodium, it is important that we read and understand food labels. For example, 0.5g sodium and over per 100g of food is considered high in salt and 0.1g of sodium or less is considered low in salt. Starchy carbohydrates and fruits and vegetables are naturally low in salt. Cutting down on salt can help to lower our blood pressure. Eating God's way means that we would be consuming a diet low in salt anyway!

Chapter VI

FLUID CONSUMPTION

Two thirds of our body consists of water so it is our most important nutrient. In fact, water is more crucial than food because we can survive without food for approximately 30-40 days but only 3-5 days without water. This is because water is involved in almost every bodily process – digestion, absorption, circulation (delivery and transport) and excretion.

We should be consuming at least 1 litre of water a day, ideally our fluid intake should be 2 litres a day as we lose on average, approximately 1.5 litres, daily, through our skin, lungs, digestive system and kidneys. It is important therefore that this lost water is replaced on a daily basis. Aim to drink at least a litre of water, daily. If possible avoid drinking tap water or at the very least, filter it to remove any impurities. Spring, distilled or filtered water are good options because they contain a limited amount of impurities.

Living Water!
Did you know that dehydration slows your metabolism, is the number one cause of daytime fatigue, back pain and joint pain, affects memory, focus and vision and has been associated with an increased risk of certain cancers such as colon, breast and bladder?

A word about juices

To further increase our fluid intake, drinking fruit or vegetable juices (i.e. freshly squeezed/blended home made varieties rather than the processed, high sugar varieties from the supermarkets) is a good way to nourish, detoxify and hydrate our cells. Fruit and vegetable juices help to hydrate the body, provide a natural source of sugar, fibre, vitamins and minerals and other goodies that the body was designed to run on. Fruit and vegetable juices that have been processed tend to be high in added sugar – and may contain other substances such as preservatives, artificial colours and flavours that the body was not designed to process. If you cannot avoid the high sugar processed varieties in the supermarkets, dilute them with the same quantity of water. Aim to drink 2 litres of fluid a day in the form of water, fresh juices, herbal or fruit teas, natural tea and coffee alternatives. Home made juices drunk soon after preparation are the best and most nutritious, therefore investing in a blender or juicer is a good idea.

Drink Up!
Fruit and vegetables are made up of approximately 90% water and can therefore contribute to our daily fluid intake.

Carbonated drinks

Artificially carbonated water and drinks have been associated with depleting natural mineral levels in the body. In addition, many fizzy drinks are very high in processed sugars, sweeteners, colourings, preservatives and additives.

Tea, Coffee and Alcohol

Our body was not designed to run on or process concentrated amounts of stimulants. Consistent consumption of stimulants such as tea, coffee and alcohol cause the body to lose water - because they act as diuretics - and rob our body of essential nutrients at the same time. Stimulants like tea, coffee and alcohol also cause blood sugar levels to rise and fall rapidly leading to negative emotions such as irritability, anxiety, and depression, and over-eating.

In addition, these substances are addictive. It is therefore wise to avoid them where possible. The negative effects of consuming them far outweigh the benefits. If you think you can't do without them in your diet you may have an addiction, or you may have made the substance an 'idol'. Avoid or greatly reduce your intake of tea, coffee and alcohol. Of course, the best prevention is to avoid these stimulants completely.

More on Alcohol

There is much debate and division in the Christian community with regards to the consumption of alcohol. In the Bible, there is reference to alcohol being used for medicinal purposes;

> *No longer drink only water but use a little wine for your stomach's sake and your frequent infirmities.*
>
> 1 Timothy 5:23,

And also some positive reference to alcohol in certain places in the Scriptures for example, Ecclesiastes 9:7a and 10:19

> *Go eat your bread with joy and drink your wine with a merry heart*
>
> Ecclesiastes 9:7a

> *A feast is made for laughter, and wine makes merry*
>
> Ecclesiastes 9:7a

There are also numerous occasions in Scripture where restrictions are placed on the consumption of alcohol and where warnings of its negative effects are given. For example, for those serving as priests, the following advice was given;

> *Do not drink wine or intoxicating drink, you, nor your sons with you, when you go into the tabernacle of meeting, lest you die. It shall be a statute forever throughout your generations.*
>
> Leviticus 10:9

For those taking the vow of a Nazarite, the advice was even stricter;

> *He shall separate himself from wine and similar drink; he shall drink neither vinegar made from wine nor vinegar made from similar drink; neither shall he drink any grape juice, nor eat fresh grapes or raisins.*
>
> Numbers 6:3,

Other Scriptures state the following truths about alcohol;

> *Wine is a mocker, strong drink is a brawler, and whoever is led astray by it is not wise.*
>
> Proverbs 20:1,

> *It is not for kings, O Lemuel. It is not for kings to drink wine, nor for princes intoxicating drink; lest they drink and forget the law and pervert the justice of all the afflicted. Give strong drink to him who is perishing, and wine to those who are bitter of heart. Let him drink and forget his poverty, and remember his misery no more.*

Proverbs 31:4-7

Who has woe? Who has sorrow? Who has contentions? Who has complaints? Who has wounds without cause? Who has redness of eyes? Those who linger long at the wine, those who go in search of mixed wine. Do not look on the wine when it is red, and sparkles in the cup, when it swirls around smoothly; at the last it bites like a serpent, and stings like a viper. Your eyes will see strange things, and your heart will utter perverse things. Yes, you will be like one who lies down in the midst of the sea or like one who lies at the top of the mast saying "They have struck me, but I was not hurt; they have beaten me, but I did not feel it. When shall I awake that I may seek another drink?"

Proverbs 23:29-35

I honestly doubt the primary reason many drink alcohol is for medicinal purposes! But rather for pleasure and recreation. Christians are cautioned to be filled with the Holy Spirit and not with wine.

And do not be drunk with wine, in which is dissipation; but be filled with the Spirit.

Ephesians 5:18

Many use Jesus as an example, stating that He consumed alcohol and clearly Jesus is our example and thus the logic of this is understandable. However, in ancient times, the alcoholic content of such drinks was limited to the amount of alcohol produced by the natural fermentation process which stops naturally when about 11% to 14% of the juice is alcohol. However due to the later widespread advent of the artificial manufacturing process of distillation – A.D. 500 - the percentage of alcohol is by far higher in many of the hard liquors and spirits we see today than in the "strong drink" referred to in biblical times. In fact, distilled alcoholic beverages such as whiskey, gin, vodka and rum can contain 40% - 50% alcohol.

Thus, the more potent fortified and distilled alcoholic beverages we see today are not the same as the wine and strong drink referred to in the Bible. Even if we were to say that "pleasurable" alcohol consumption is not prohibited in the Bible, and only excess and drunkenness are cautioned, we could still safely conclude that consuming the potent modern day varieties of alcohol fortified through distillation is not what Scripture advocates.

Needless to say, alcohol is not an essential nutrient required by the body. Looking at some of the negative effects that are associated with alcohol consumption such as depression of the central nervous system, lack of judgement and co-ordination, suppression of the immune system, increased blood pressure, blocking of nutrient absorption, birth defects, mental defects and addictive habit forming capacity (not to talk of the social effects of family breakdown and violence associated with addiction) it is clear to see why the substance would be best avoided.

If we take the whole picture into account, there are

more reasons to avoid alcohol altogether than there are to drink it. It really doesn't make sense to pour a chemical with such high evidence of habit-forming activity associated with such negative effects into our bodies - after all, we are the temple of the Living God.

It is also true that as ambassadors for Jesus we have given up our rights to live only for ourselves. Romans 14:21 says that

> *It is good neither to eat meat nor drink wine, nor do anything by which your brother stumbles or is offended or is made weak.*
>
> Romans 14:21

Thus for the sake of the gospel, it may be necessary to avoid alcohol. Of course, it's really down to one's personal convictions on the matter, however the best form of prevention is always total abstinence!

A Final Word on Tea, Coffee and Alcohol

Tea and coffee contain the natural plant substance, caffeine. Alcohol is actually a by-product of the natural fermentation of fruit and is also natural. However, in large amounts, caffeine and alcohol can exhibit stimulant, addictive and habit-forming activity on the body. Caffeine is found in tea and coffee but also in a host of foods you may not suspect like dairy products and chocolate, cola, and cocoa. Stimulants such as caffeine and alcohol in concentrated amounts, or if consistently consumed over time have been linked with psychological problems, behavioural problems, teratogenicity, dehydration, poor judgement, cancer and heart conditions.

Chapter VII

FOOD PREPARATION & THE USE OF SUPPLEMENTS

Food Preparation Methods

It is imperative to eat a healthy balanced diet to maintain good health; however it is equally important to pay attention to how the food is prepared. Food must be prepared in such a way as to conserve nutrients as best as possible and also to avoid the formation of harmful substances. For example, cooking food to browning or charring encourages the formation of harmful cancer causing substances called carcinogens.

In order to retain the goodness of the foods we eat, a

combination of the following cooking methods may be employed:

- Steaming - where the food is cooked in steam from boiling water or from the food itself, in which case it is within a container surrounded by steam or boiling water.

- Roasting/baking - Where the food is cooked by dry heat in an oven.

- Poaching - a very similar method to boiling however the liquid does not bubble and the food is just only submerged. The temperature is just below boiling point.

- Grilling - a high-heat cooking method done directly over or under live flames, cooking the food in a matter of minutes

Avoid or greatly reduce frying of any sort as this method produces potentially harmful compounds called free radicals that can damage our body's cells thus increasing diseases such as cancer, heart disease, premature ageing as well as destroying essential nutrients meant to protect us from such damage.

There are also other considerations we need to bear in mind when planning and preparing our meals.

- Eat raw/natural food where possible – particularly fruit and vegetables, seeds and nuts.

- Eat organic or chemically free produce - at the very least, thoroughly wash/scrub fruit and vegetables to minimise the amount of chemical residues entering the body. Some health food stores sell non-toxic rinsing preparations that can equally be used for rinsing.

- Eat free-range products where possible.
- Eat Kosher products – Kosher food is food prepared in accordance with Jewish dietary guidelines or 'Kashrut' which means proper. It does not mean, as many tend to think, that it has been offered to idols. Kosher meat and poultry are slaughtered under strict guidelines called 'shechita' i.e. slaughtered without pain, inspected for illness, abnormalities and anything else that is considered harmful or unhygienic. The lungs must be pure and all the fat and blood is removed.

Food Supplements

I do not believe it was ever God's initial intention for us to need or take supplements. Unfortunately things are not the same now as they were back in the Garden of Eden. For a start, back in Adam and Eve's day, food was not exposed to the extensive processing it is now, neither was it subject to the addition of various artificial substances such as preservatives, additives, flavours and colours.

For most of us, eating a healthy, balanced diet will provide us with all the necessary nutrients for health and well-being. However, the key question is, how many of us are consuming a healthy, balanced, diet on a consistent basis?

Indeed nutritional supplements may be recommended and beneficial in certain circumstances. For example, during pregnancy or for individuals who omit entire food groupings from their diet such as vegetarians and vegans, or those with intolerances or allergies. Supplements may also be required during illness and convalescence or for medical reasons. Your doctor or dietician may advise you of your personal vitamin and mineral requirements and whether or not you are deficient in certain nutrients.

Supplementing Your Meal

Taking supplements with meals helps to ensure a supply of other nutrients which are needed for better assimilation. Do follow the dose and instructions and remember to consult your doctor before taking supplements.

Supplements can come in many forms, for example tablets, capsules, lozenges, liquid formulations, and injections. There are so many on the market these days, and with such an array and so many claims of benefit, it can be quite confusing and overwhelming at times to decide which to choose .

If you feel you will benefit from taking a multivitamin and mineral supplement, it's probably best to start by selecting supplements on what you really need. And do not be afraid to ask the pharmacist for help if you require it. As a rule, avoid supplements with high dose single vitamins or minerals, as they may not really be necessary. Also supplements can be harmful in high doses. In fact, you may find a supplement that contains several of the nutrients needed in one tablet or capsule which is probably more cost effective and beneficial. However, always remember to consult your doctor. Your doctor is aware of your full medical history and is thus in a better position to advise you. Also remember that supplements are exactly what they say they are – supplements. Their purpose is to *supplement* the diet, not to *substitute* it. Supplements can never replace a healthy, balanced, varied diet.

Chapter VIII

FASTING

According to the Webster's Dictionary, fasting is defined as "abstaining from food" or "the act of abstaining from food". Some religions assign certain days or periods for fasting, such as Lent and Ramadan. In reality we all fast naturally every night when we go to sleep, and we break-the-fast when we take our 'breakfast' in the morning.

When the Bible talks of fasting however, it is talking about much more than just the abstinence from food. Abstaining from food is just a part of the biblical fast and it is imperative that we understand this. Indeed God rebuked the Israelites for abusing the fast and we certainly don't want to make the same mistakes. The biblical fast is a powerful sacrificial adjunct to prayer that produces results. Thus we need to be clear whether we are referring to the biblical fast, or whether we are simply referring to abstinence from food when we talk about "fasting".

The Physical Perspective

Abstaining from food may have beneficial effects on the body in some individuals. By abstaining from food(s) we are, in effect, giving the body a rest from certain foods and/or drinks. During the abstinence period, we may also rid the body of excess toxins that can accumulate due to what we eat. By reducing the amount of food we eat, the body will spend less energy digesting food and can thus channel that energy into other body processes such as detoxification and immunity. Thus abstaining from certain foodstuffs may help cleanse the body and eliminate toxic or harmful substances that may have been causing aggravation, and possibly ill health.

Important Advice

Should you wish to start a fasting program for health reasons, it is imperative that you seek medical supervision and advice prior to commencing. Your GP should be informed of any sudden changes in dietary pattern prior to it happening. Women who are pregnant or considering pregnancy, have any form of chronic illness such as diabetes, kidney or liver disease should not abstain from food without the consent of their medical practitioner.

Abstinence may also assist in some level of weight loss, reduce the severity and incidence of certain diseases and enhance overall health and well-being.

Some individuals have reported reductions in cholesterol levels, blood pressure, inflammation and joint pain, loss of weight, mental benefits including increased clarity, focus and concentration and relief from addictions as a result of fasting. However, these health benefits can also be achieved by eating a healthy, balanced diet.

The Spiritual Perspective

God's definition of fasting is very different to man's. For a start, God's fasting is based on spiritual principles. Let's not be disillusioned here – the fast that God talks about is more than abstinence from food.

According to the Bible, prayer should accompany fasting. Indeed, on further examination of the Scriptures, there are also crucial conditions to the fast that go far beyond mere abstinence from food and drink. For example, it may include sharing food with the hungry, helping the homeless and naked, and doing away with backbiting and slandering. Thus, true fasting is about one's heart attitude as well as the act of self-denial.

When I examined some of the scriptures on fasting, I found that one of the similarities between the texts was that the individuals who were fasting were also seeking God in some way. That is to say, they were using the act of abstinence as an adjunct to some form of prayer. Let's take for example the prophet Ezra. In Ezra chapter 8 verses 21 through to 23, we see that Ezra called a nationwide fast in order to seek God for an answer;

> *Then I proclaimed a fast there at the river of Ahava, that we might humble ourselves before our God, to seek from Him the right way for us and our little ones and all our possessions. For I was ashamed to request of the king an escort of soldiers and horsemen to help us against the enemy on the road, because we had spoken to the king saying, "The hand of our God is upon all those for good who seek Him, but His power and His wrath are against all those who forsake Him." So we fasted and entreated our God for this, and He answered our prayer.*
>
> Ezra 8:21-23

Thus not only did Ezra fast, but he also prayed.

Or take the prophet Daniel who also practiced the biblical fast.

> *Then I set my face toward the Lord God to make request by prayer and supplications, with fasting, sackcloth, and ashes.*
>
> Daniel 9:3

Notice Daniel, like Ezra used fasting as an adjunct to prayer. The last thing on the minds of these men of God was whether or not their cholesterol levels were going to be reduced or whether they were going to reach their target weight! In fact, it would be true to say that these men were already consuming the diet prescribed by their Creator and thus the emphasis of the fast didn't need to be for health reasons.

The biblical fast, used in its proper context is indeed a powerful tool in the Christian's life and should never be abused or confused with mere self-denial. Yes, it involves the discipline of denial of nourishment, but this must be coupled with prayer and seeking the Lord during that abstinence.

For more clarity, let's look again at Scripture and compare fasting to abstinence. The well-known story of Daniel is a very good example of self-denial;

> *But Daniel purposed in his heart that he would not defile himself with the portion of the king's delicacies, nor with the wine which he drank; therefore he requested of the chief of the eunuchs that he might not defile himself. Now God had brought Daniel into the favour and goodwill of the chief of the eunuchs. And the chief of the eunuchs said to Daniel, "I fear for my lord the king, who has appointed your food and drink. For why should he see your faces looking worse than the young men who are your age? Then you would endanger my head before the king." So Daniel said to the steward whom the chief of the eunuchs had set over Daniel, Hananiah, Mishael and Azariah, "Please test your servants for ten days, and let them give us vegetables to eat and eater to drink. Then let our appearance be examined before you, and the appearance of the young men who eat the portion of the king's*

delicacies; and as you see fit, so deal with your servants." So he consented with them in this matter, and tested them ten days. And at the end of the ten days their features appeared better and fatter in flesh than all the young men who ate the portion of the king's delicacies. Thus the steward took away their portion of delicacies and the wine that they were to drink and gave them vegetables.

Daniel 1:8-16

We are not told of what the king's delicacies were, but Daniel and his friends chose to be disciplined and not consume them. It is possible that these delicacies included substances that God had not prescribed in His original diet, and Daniel and his friends were therefore showing both discipline and obedience. In fact, to Daniel and his friends, abstaining from the king's delicacies was probably not viewed as abstinence of any sort – it was probably their natural way of life and dietary habits.

Whatever the case, the point of this story is that it shows not only the physical benefits of abstaining from certain food ingredients, but more importantly the difference between abstinence and the biblical fast discussed above in the previous examples of Ezra and Daniel.

If we examine Isaiah 58:6-12 in a little more detail we not only see the conditions God requires for the fasting He desires, but also we can see the spiritual benefits of such a fast;

Is this not the fast that I have chosen? To loose the bonds of wickedness, to undo the heavy burdens, to let the oppressed go free, and that you break every yoke? Is it not to share your bread with the hungry, and that you bring to your house the poor who are cast out. When you see the naked, that you cover him; and not hide yourself from your own flesh? Then your light shall break forth like the morning, your healing shall spring forth speedily, and your righteousness shall go before you; the glory of the Lord shall be your rear guard. Then you shall call and the Lord will answer; you shall cry and He will say "Here I am". If you take away the yoke from your midst, the pointing of your finger, and speaking wickedness. If you extend your soul to the hungry and satisfy the afflicted soul, then your light shall dawn in the darkness, and your darkness shall be as the noonday; the Lord will guide thee continually, and satisfy your soul in drought, and strengthen your bones: you shall be like a watered garden, and like a spring of water, whose waters do not fail. Those from among you shall build the old waste places: you shall raise up the foundations of many generations and you shall be called the Repairer of the Breach, The Restorer of Streets to Dwell in.

Isaiah 58:6-12

Thus, the primary purpose and rewards of the biblical fast are undeniably spiritual. Jesus' teaching further encourages us to pray, fast, give alms and forgive.

There are typically three different types of fast that we are familiar with;

a) The **normal fast** - not eating food for a definite time period. An example of this type of fast is given in Luke chapter 4 verses 1 to 2;

> *Then Jesus, being filled with the Holy Spirit, returned from the Jordan and was led by the Spirit into the wilderness, being tempted for forty days by the devil. And in those days He ate nothing, and afterward, when they had ended, He was hungry.*
>
> Luke 4:1-2

b) The **absolute fast** - not eating food or drinking water. This really should be shorter than the normal fast. This is because your body cannot go without water for longer than three to four days. This fast would have to be divinely inspired. Moses undertook such as fast and Deuteronomy chapter 9 verse 18 details it for us;

> *And I fell down before the Lord, as at the first, forty days and forty nights; I neither ate bread nor drank water, because of all your sin which you committed in doing wickedly in the sight of the Lord, to provoke Him to anger.*
>
> Deuteronomy 9:18

c) The **partial fast -** includes omitting one meal a day, or certain foods for a period of time. Some cite Daniel's example as an illustration of a partial fast. However Daniel's choice not to eat the king's delicacies may have been a lifestyle for him and his friends rather than a fast in the sense of abstaining from certain foods for a period of time.

Whatever the case we should endeavour to make fasting a part of our Christian walk rather than a one-off exercise. The Bible states "when you fast", not "if you fast" (Matthew 6:16). We should really incorporate fasting as part of our Christian lifestyle.

However, we are also to ensure that it is divinely inspired and done with wisdom. Whatever you do, make sure your motives are right. The Biblical fast is for seeking the Lord. Don't go into it with the motive of loosing weight - that would be a weight loss program or health regime, not true fasting. Indeed you may find you reap some physical benefits. However, to reap the full benefits of the Biblical fast it must be done with a pure motive and sincere heart, and must be coupled with prayer and good works.

Chapter IX

CONCLUDING WORDS

God loves us. He created our physical bodies and knows what is best and necessary for it to function optimally for His highest glory. His dietary principles are not burdensome, but are designed to ensure that we consume a wholesome diet. The Creator's diet is food high in fibre, low in fat, animal protein and cholesterol. It also contains many ingredients that help prevent illness and bring healing at the same time. The interesting thing is that nutritionists and health professionals all over the world are slowly coming round to God's way of thinking concerning physical health.

Don't be too hard on yourself

Your appetite, tastes and dietary choices are what they are because of what you are accustomed to. It takes a lifetime to develop unhealthy eating habits and it will take God's grace and your total commitment to obey Him to change to His way. When you begin to change your diet in obedience to your Creator it is likely to be difficult initially (you may even stumble a few times) but if you stay the course, eventually you will begin to get used to it and even begin to enjoy it. You will also enjoy the additional benefit of good health.

Take one day at a time and do what you know to be right. Don't be too hard on yourself. I encourage you to go for it, you can do it. The Bible affirms this;

> I can do all things through Christ who strengthens me.
>
> Philippians 4:13

God's principles WORK and they don't change from day-to-day but are the same yesterday, today and forever. Our part of the covenant is to listen and consistently obey Him. Remember these important principles:

- Eat only what our loving Father calls food.
- Eat food in it's most natural state before it has been tampered with or refined by humans into what they think is best for us.
- Eat a variety of the foods.
- Don't let food become your idol or god – avoid substances that are addictive.

- Enjoy healthy eating.
- Enjoy healthy living.

When we take these principles, together with regular exercise, fresh air, sunshine, faith, hope, and prayer, we will be well on our way to reaping many health rewards.

Sometimes God may choose to heal supernaturally, however He doesn't always do so. He may choose to bring healing to us through natural means, such as healthy eating, exercise etc. As a result we need to start taking responsibility for our health, using the principles and provisions He has made available to us in His Word. His Word is life and health to all who find them.

If you have truly surrendered your heart to God, and acknowledge that He is Master in your life, then out of faithful obedience and love, you will have pleasure in surrendering your entire life to His way – even down to your eating habits!

BIBLIOGRAPHY

i.   What the Bible says about healthy living. Rex Russel M.D. Regal Books. Health and Nutrition 1996.

ii. Eden's Health Plan – Go Natural. Mark and Patti Virkler 1994.

iii. The Optimum Nutrition Bible. Patrick Holford. Founder of the Institute for Optimum Nutrition 1997.

iv. What does the Bible teach about clean and unclean meats? United Church of God – An International Association. David Treybig, 2001.

v.   The Soil Association www.soilassociation.org 2002-2006

vi. Back to Eden – Classic Guide to Herbal Medicine, Natural Food and Home Remedies since 1939. Jethro Kloss 1991.

vii. The Maker's Diet, Jordan S Rubin 2004.

viii. Prescription for Nutritional Healing – A practical A-Z Reference to Drug-Free Remedies Using Vitamins, Minerals, Herbs and Food Supplements. Third Edition. Phyllis A Balch, James F Balch 2000

ix. Beer and Wine: The Bible's Counsel. Signs of the Times 115:2-4 William H Shea 1988a.

x.   Fermentation versus distillation. Louis Rushmore 2001. www.gospelgazette.com

xi. Manual of Dietetic Practice. 3rd Ed. Bryony Thomas in conjunction with the British Dietetic Association 2001.

Food Standards Agency – www.food.gov.uk

APPENDIX 1: VITAMINS AND MINERALS

VITAMIN	FUNCTION	EXAMPLES OF FOOD SOURCES
Vitamin A (Retinol and beta-carotene)	Helps maintain healthy skin and mucous membranes (e.g. the nose), helps vision and strengthens immunity from infections	Dairy foods, liver, fish liver oils, carrots, yellow, orange and green vegetables
Vitamin B1 (Thiamin)	Release of energy from food, and helps keep nerve and muscle tissue healthy	Poultry, fish and beans, vegetables, milk, cheese, peas, fresh and dried fruit, wholegrain breads and some fortified breakfast cereals
Vitamin B2 (Riboflavin)	Helps keep skin, eyes and mucous membranes healthy, helps produce steroids and red blood cells and may help the body absorb iron from the food we eat	Milk, eggs, rice and mushrooms, fortified breakfast cereals
Niacin	Helps release energy from the foods we eat and helps keep the nervous and digestive system healthy	Beef, chicken, wheat flour, maize flour, eggs and milk

VITAMIN	FUNCTION	EXAMPLES OF FOOD SOURCES
Vitamin B6 (pyridoxine)	Allows the body to use and store the energy from the foods we eat, and helps form haemoglobin (the substance that carries oxygen around the body)	Chicken, turkey, cod, bread, whole grains (such as oatmeal, wheatgerm and rice), eggs, vegetables, soya beans, peanuts, milk, potatoes and some fortified breakfast cereals
Vitamin B12	Helps release energy from the foods we eat, helps keep the nervous system healthy and make red blood cells, needed to process folic acid	Virtually all meat products, and algae such as seaweed, meat, salmon, cod, milk, cheese, eggs, yeast extract, and some fortified breakfast cereals
Folate	Works with B12 to make red blood cells and reduces the risk of neural tube defects in new born babies	Broccoli and Brussels sprouts, peas, chick peas, yeast extract, brown rice and some fruits (such as bananas and oranges). Also bread and some fortified breakfast cereals

VITAMIN	FUNCTION	EXAMPLES OF FOOD SOURCES
Pantothenic Acid	Helps release energy from the foods we eat	Virtually all vegetables and meat, chicken, beef, potatoes, porridge, tomatoes, kidney, egg, broccoli and whole grains such as wholemeal bread and brown rice
Vitamin C	Helps protect cells and keeps them healthy, and helps absorb iron from foods	Found in a wide variety of fruit and vegetables such as peppers, broccoli, oranges and kiwi fruit, sweet potatoes, Brussels sprouts
Vitamin D	Helps regulate the amount of calcium and phosphate in the body which are important for healthy bones and teeth	Oily fish, eggs and fortified foods such as margarine, breakfast cereals, bread
Vitamin E	Antioxidant properties help to protect cells	Soya, corn and olive oils, nuts, seeds and wheatgerm (found in cereals and their products)
Vitamin K	Helps wounds heal properly and helps to build strong bones	Broccoli, spinach and vegetable oils, and cereals, meat and cheese

VITAMIN	FUNCTION	EXAMPLES OF FOOD SOURCES
Biotin	Helps release/turn food into energy	Meat, kidney, eggs, fruit and vegetables including dried fruit

MINERAL/ TRACE ELEMENT	FUNCTION	EXAMPLES OF FOOD SOURCES
Sodium	Helps to keep the levels of fluid in the body in balance	Found naturally in all foods at low levels but very high amounts are found in processed foods such as processed meats and meat products, condiments, sauces and gravies
Chloride	Helps to keep the levels of fluid in the body in balance and helps the body digest the food we eat because it is a component of the digestive juices	Sea weed, soy sauce, rye
Calcium	Helps to build strong bones and teeth, regulates muscle contraction including the heartbeat and makes sure blood clots normally	Milk and dairy products such as yogurt and cheeses, green leafy vegetables such as broccoli and cabbage and fish bones (sardines, pilchards)

MINERAL/ TRACE ELEMENT	FUNCTION	EXAMPLES OF FOOD SOURCES
Phosphorus	Like calcium, helps to build strong bones and teeth, and helps to release energy from the food we eat	Red meat, dairy products, rice and oats, bread, fish and poultry
Potassium	Controls the balance of fluids in the body and is involved in the lowering of blood pressure	Fruit (bananas), vegetables, pulses, avocado, nuts and seeds, white meat and fish
Chromium	Helps to regulate blood sugar levels	Meat, whole grains, lentils and spices
Copper	Helps to produce red and white blood cells, and triggers the release of iron to form haemoglobin – the substance that carries oxygen around the body	Nuts, almonds, avocados, beans, broccoli, lentils, oranges, soybeans, green leafy vegetables and salmon
Iodine	Helps to make the thyroid hormones which regulate our body's metabolism	Cereals and grains and cow's milk (in the UK)

MINERAL/ TRACE ELEMENT	FUNCTION	EXAMPLES OF FOOD SOURCES
Iron	Helps to make red blood cells which carry oxygen around the body	Liver, dried fruit (such as apricots), whole grains, meat, legumes, nuts, dark green leafy vegetables, fortified breakfast cereals
Magnesium	Helps turn the food we eat into energy and for healthy bones	Green leafy vegetables and nuts, bread, fish, meat and dairy products
Manganese	Helps make and activate some enzymes in the body	Breads, nuts, cereals, green vegetables (such as peas and runner beans)
Fluoride	Contributes to the formation of strong teeth and increases resistance to tooth decay	Fish, drinking water
Molybdenum	Helps to make and activate some enzymes in the body and involved in making genetic material	Peas, leafy vegetables (including broccoli and spinach), nuts and cereals such as oats

MINERAL/ TRACE ELEMENT	FUNCTION	EXAMPLES OF FOOD SOURCES
Selenium	Plays an important part in the functioning of the immune system, and in thyroid hormone metabolism. Anti-oxidant functions – preventing damage to cells and tissues	Meat, fish and nuts
Zinc	Helps to make new cells and enzymes, helps with the healing of wounds, and helps the body process the food we eat	Meat, milk and dairy foods, bread and cereal products such a wheatgerm

APPENDIX 2: PHYTONUTRIENTS

FOOD	PHYTONUTRIENT	HEALTH ASSOCIATIONS
Garlics, onions, leeks, shallots, chives	Allium compounds	Immune and anti-cancer properties
Citrus fruits, berries, brocolli, rosehips, buckwheat leaves, cherries, grapes, papaya, canteloupe melon, plums, tomatoes, cucumber	Bioflavanoids	Binding and conducting any waste products and toxins from the body, antibiotic effects on the body, anti-infection properties, anti-cancer properties. Also involved in dealing with capillary fragility - bleeding gums, varicose veins, hemorrhoids, bruises, strain injuries, thrombosis
Hot peppers	Capsaicin	Helps protect your body's cells from damage
Wheat grass, algae, seaweed, green vegetables	Chlorophyll – the substance that makes green plants green	Helps to keep the blood healthy, anti-cancer properties, antibiotic properties

FOOD	PHYTONUTRIENT	HEALTH ASSOCIATIONS
A variety of fruit and vegetables including tomatoes ,green peppers, pineapples, strawberries and carrots	Coumarins and chlorogenic acid	Prevents the formation of cancer causing substances in the body
Strawberries, grapes, raspberries	Ellagic acid	Neutralises cancer causing substances in the body
Soya beans	Genistein	Prevents various cancers from growing and spreading.
Broccoli, Brussels sprouts, cabbage, cauliflower, cress, horseradish, kale, turnips	Isothiocyanates and Indoles	Anti-cancer properties,

FOOD	PHYTONUTRIENT	HEALTH ASSOCIATIONS
Soya (tofu and miso), pulses (beans, peas), citrus fruits, alfalfa, fennel and celery	Phytoestrogens	Anti-cancer properties
Broccoli, cauliflower, Brussels sprouts, turnips, kale	Sulforaphane	Reduces the risk of breast cancer

Adapted from The Optimum Nutrition Bible. Patrick Holford – founder of the Institute for Optimum Nutrition.

APPENDIX 3: CLEAN (HEALTHY) AND UNCLEAN (UNHEALTHY) ANIMALS

The Clean (Healthy)
Animals that chew the cud and part the hoof
Antelope, buffalo, caribou, cattle (beef, veal), deer (venison), elk, gazelle, giraffe, goat, hart, ibex, moose, ox, reindeer, sheep (lamb, mutton).

Fish with fins and scales
Anchovy, barracuda, bass, black pomfret (monchong), bluefish, bluegill, carp, cod, crappie, drum, flounder, grouper, grunt, haddock, hake, halibut, hardhead, herring, kingfish, mackerel, dolphin fish, minnow, mullet, bream, pike, Pollock, rockfish, salmon, sardine (pilchard), shad, silver hake (whiting), smelt, snapper, sole, steelhead, sucker, sunfish, tarpon, trout, tuna, whitefish.

Birds with clean characteristics
Chicken, dove, duck, goose, grouse, guinea fowl, partridge, peafowl, pheasant, pigeon (wood), prarie, ptarmigan, quail, sage hen, sparrow (and other songbirds), swan, teal, turkey.

Insects
Types of locusts that may include crickets and grasshoppers.

The Unclean (Unhealthy)
Swine
Boar, peaccary, pig (hog, bacon, ham, lard, pork, most sausage and pepperoni).

Canines
Coyote, dog, fox, hyena, jackal, wolf.

Felines
Cat, cheetah, leopard, lion, panther, tiger.

Equines
Ass, donkey, horse, mule, onager, zebra.

Other
Armidillo, badger, bear, beaver, camel, elephant, gorilla, groundhog, hare, hippopotamus, kangaroo, llama, mole, monkey, mouse, muskrat, opossum, porcupine, rabbit, raccoon, rat, rhinocerous, skunk, slug, snail, squirrel, wallaby, weasel, wolverine, worm.

Insects
All insects except some in the locust family.

Marine animals without scales and fins
Fish: bullhead, catfish, eel, European turbot, marlin, paddlefish, sculpin, shark, stickleback, squid, sturgeon (includes most caviar), swordfish.

Shellfish: abalone, clam, crab, crayfish, lobster, mussel,

prawn, oyster, scallop, shrimp.

Soft body: cuttlefish, jellyfish, limpet, octopus, squid (calamari).

Sea Mammals: dolphin, otter, porpoise, seal, walrus, whale.

Birds of prey, scavengers and others
Albatross, bat, bittern, buzzard, condor, coot, cormorant, crane, crow, cuckoo, eagle, flamingo, grebe, grosbeak, gull, hawk, heron, kite, lapwing, loon, magpie, osprey, ostrich, owl, parrot, pelican, penguin, plover, rail, raven, roadrunner, sandpiper, seagull, stork, swallow, swift, vulture, water hen, woodpecker.

Reptiles
Alligator, caiman, crocodile, lizard, snake, turtle.

Amphibians
Blindworm, frog, newt, salamander, toad.

APPENDIX 4: SAMPLE 4-DAY EATING PLAN

This is by no means a rigid plan, but illustrates and gives a general idea of how healthy eating can be incorporated into the day. It may take a little preparation in advance but the health benefits are really worth the effort.

Day 1

BREAKFAST One serving of old fashioned porridge oats with semi-skimmed milk topped with 2 tablespoons fruit (e.g. raisins, berries, sliced almonds, walnuts); one medium glass of freshly blended juice or a portion of a fruit of your choice e.g. pear.

LUNCH One medium-sized jacket potato/sweet potato with a little olive oil and tuna mix (tuna, onions, black pepper) served with a side salad with vinegar salad dressing (olive oil, vinegar, salt and pepper to taste).

DINNER Stir-fried chicken with vegetables (ginger, mushrooms, bamboo shoots, mange-tout, spring onions, sesame oil) served with a small serving of brown or basmati rice; bowl of fruit salad with live yogurt pot.

Day 2

BREAKFAST Scrambled eggs on wholemeal toast with grilled tomatoes; one medium glass of freshly squeezed/blended juice or portion of a fruit of your choice e.g. half a grapefruit.

LUNCH One wholemeal pitta pocket with sliced turkey and raw peppers, shredded romaine lettuce and cherry tomatoes; one portion of fruit of your choice e.g. peach.

DINNER Steamed fish fillet e.g. cod, red bream, pollack, snapper with okra served with sweet potato and steamed carrots; fruit of choice with live yogurt pot.

Day 3

BREAKFAST Serving of wholegrain muesli with semi-skimmed milk; one medium glass of freshly squeezed/ blended juice e.g. orange juice or portion of fruit of your choice e.g. apple.

LUNCH Bowl of fresh soup e.g. lentil, vegetable, carrot and coriander served with a wholemeal, seeded roll and side salad; one portion of fruit of your choice e.g. banana.

DINNER Oven cooked fresh salmon fillet with new potatoes served with unlimited salad (vinegar salad dressing optional); mixed berries and small scoop of ice-cream.

Day 4

BREAKFAST One slice wholemeal toast with two

vegetarian soya based sausages; one glass of freshly squeezed/blended juice or one portion of fruit of your choice e.g. two small nectarines.

LUNCH Wholemeal pitta pocket with mackerel/sardines and tomatoes; fruit salad.

DINNER Chickpea curry with basmati or brown rice; homemade fruit sorbet (fresh fruit [e.g. apple, banana and pear or strawberries, banana and blueberries or mango, pear and apples or pineapple, raspberries and bananas], semi-skimmed milk, honey, blend and freeze).

NB. Watch portion sizes. Eat slowly and listen carefully to your body when it signals that it is full. Use oils sparingly and try not to add salt where possible. Instead, season with garlic, onions, challotts, black pepper, lemon and lime juice. Aim for at least 5 portions of fruit and vegetables a day and drink at least 8 glasses of fluid a day in the form of fresh fruit juices, herbal teas and water. When snacking, try and snack on fruit and vegetables, nuts and seeds – make eating fruit and vegetables a part of your every day life.

The Creator's Diet